CYCLING

A GUIDE TO MENSTRUATION

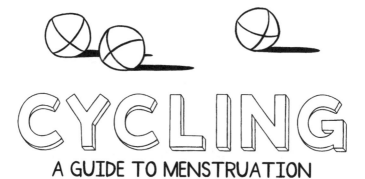

CYCLING

A GUIDE TO MENSTRUATION

Written & illustrated by

Laura Szumowski

For me when I was in the 4th grade,
because this book would have come in handy.

ISBN 978-0-9828224-2-5

LCCN 2010938820

Printed, sold and distributed with permission
by Luci Daum Design LLC.

Special thanks to all of the people who
offered their input, feedback, and
grammatical expertise.

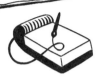 *a Note*

Knowing what's normal for your body makes you a better advocate for your own health. Being informed* keeps your body from being mysterious, and you from being uncertain. Understanding the changes you experience with your cycle informs your overall health, both physically and mentally. In other words, knowledge is power.

There is no right or wrong way to experience menstruation – every body is different. Consult a health care provider or other resources (like those at the back of this book) if you have additional questions.

*Our understanding of things like endometriosis, menstrual suppression, and dioxin is still in development, so some of this information may change.

Table of Contents

4

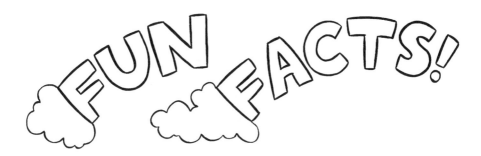

Menstruation, meaning "monthly," is often a misnomer (a wrong or innapropriate name).

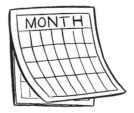

The 28-day cycle was chosen for hormonal birth control when it was first developed, so you might think it's the most natural or accurate cycle length. In actuality, healthy cycles come in a wide range of lengths.

Mittelschmerz

is a cramp or twinge that is sometimes felt in the lower abdomen or back at ovulation. About 20% of ovulators experience mittelschmerz.

As recently as the 1970s, 25% of U.S. doctors believed menstrual cramps were psychosomatic (all in your head).

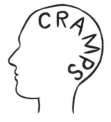

THE
menstrual
NEIGHBORHOOD

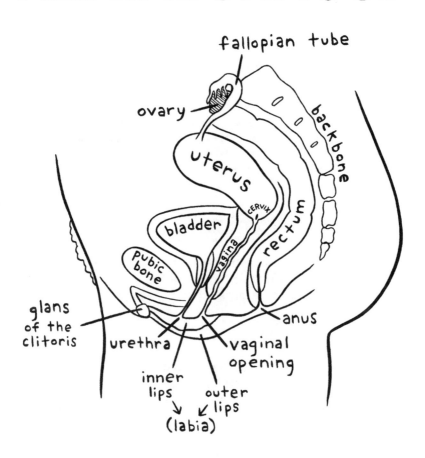

fallopian tube

ovary

backbone

uterus

bladder

CERVIX

vagina

rectum

pubic bone

glans of the clitoris

urethra

anus

vaginal opening

inner lips

outer lips

(labia)

Behold, THE Menstrual Cycle

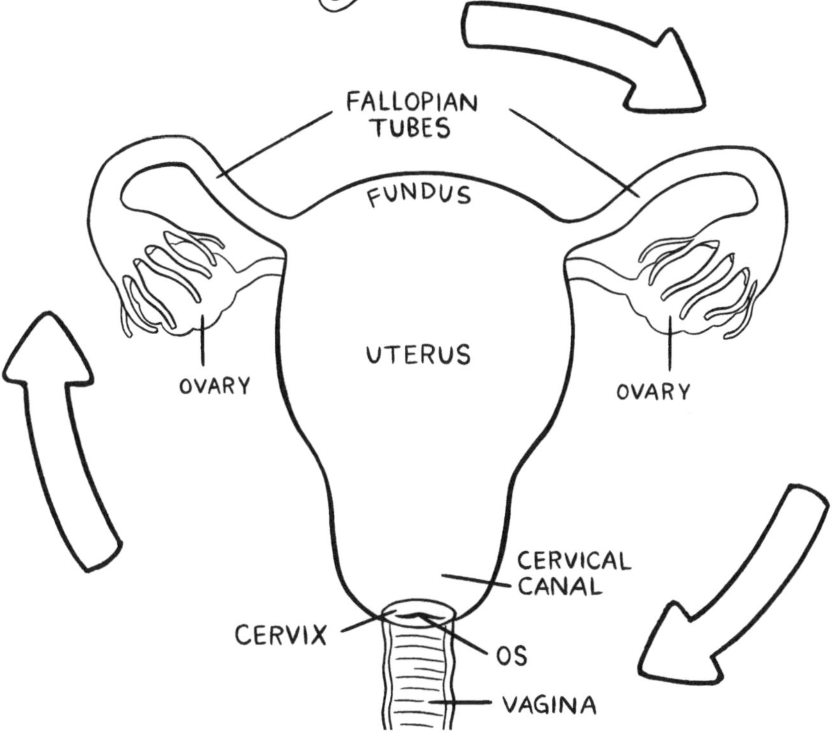

FALLOPIAN TUBES

FUNDUS

OVARY

UTERUS

OVARY

CERVICAL CANAL

CERVIX

OS

VAGINA

ovaries
⸗ featuring ⸗
FOLLICLES

OVARIES are little sacks that hold egg follicles. This is where the eggs mature, and also where hormones are produced (estrogen, progesterone, & testosterone).

A FOLLICLE is a hollow ball of cells with an egg at the center that has not yet matured.

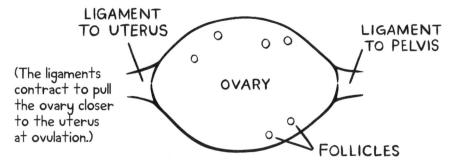

LIGAMENT TO UTERUS

LIGAMENT TO PELVIS

(The ligaments contract to pull the ovary closer to the uterus at ovulation.)

OVARY

FOLLICLES

BIRTH: ovaries contain around 2,000,000 follicles.

CHILDHOOD: ovaries absorb about HALF of the follicles.

FIRST PERIOD: there are around 400,000 – 450,000 follicles in your ovaries, ready to go.

LIFESPAN: about 300 – 500 follicles will develop into mature eggs.

8

Begin ⤵

DAY
(approx.)

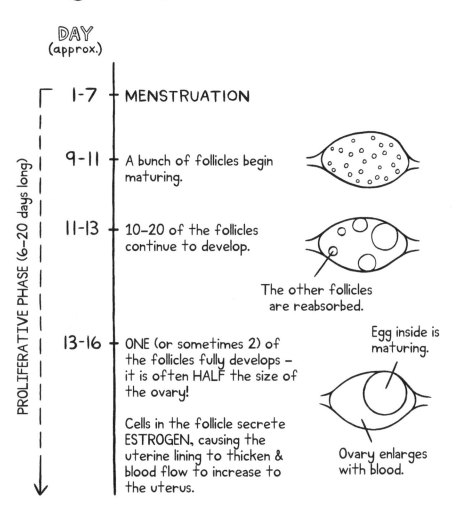

PROLIFERATIVE PHASE (6–20 days long)

1-7 — MENSTRUATION

9-11 — A bunch of follicles begin maturing.

11-13 — 10–20 of the follicles continue to develop.

The other follicles are reabsorbed.

13-16 — ONE (or sometimes 2) of the follicles fully develops – it is often HALF the size of the ovary!

Cells in the follicle secrete ESTROGEN, causing the uterine lining to thicken & blood flow to increase to the uterus.

Egg inside is maturing.

Ovary enlarges with blood.

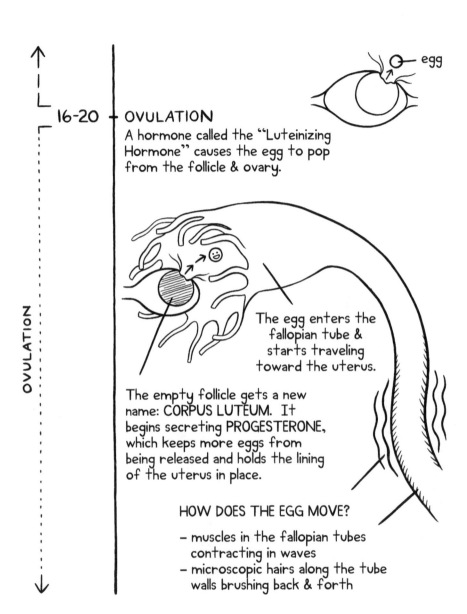

egg

16-20 — **OVULATION**
A hormone called the "Luteinizing Hormone" causes the egg to pop from the follicle & ovary.

The egg enters the fallopian tube & starts traveling toward the uterus.

The empty follicle gets a new name: CORPUS LUTEUM. It begins secreting PROGESTERONE, which keeps more eggs from being released and holds the lining of the uterus in place.

HOW DOES THE EGG MOVE?

- muscles in the fallopian tubes contracting in waves
- microscopic hairs along the tube walls brushing back & forth

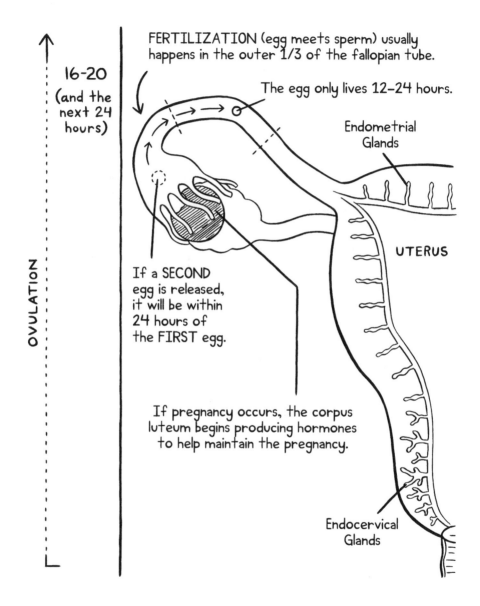

OVULATION

16-20 (and the next 24 hours)

FERTILIZATION (egg meets sperm) usually happens in the outer 1/3 of the fallopian tube.

The egg only lives 12-24 hours.

Endometrial Glands

UTERUS

If a SECOND egg is released, it will be within 24 hours of the FIRST egg.

If pregnancy occurs, the corpus luteum begins producing hormones to help maintain the pregnancy.

Endocervical Glands

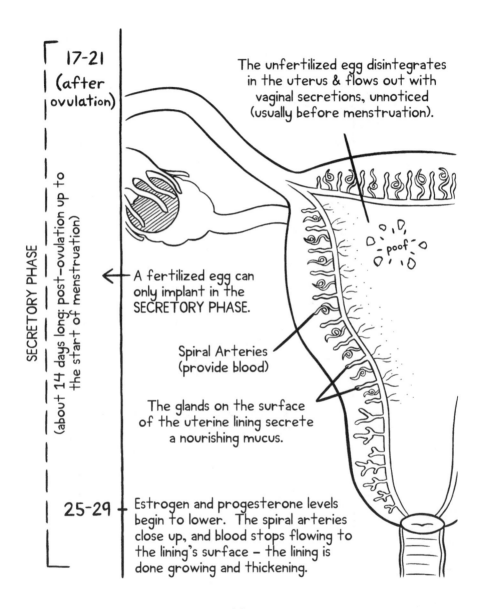

17-21
(after
ovulation)

The unfertilized egg disintegrates in the uterus & flows out with vaginal secretions, unnoticed (usually before menstruation).

SECRETORY PHASE

(about 14 days long: post-ovulation up to the start of menstruation)

← A fertilized egg can only implant in the SECRETORY PHASE.

Spiral Arteries (provide blood)

The glands on the surface of the uterine lining secrete a nourishing mucus.

poof

25-29 Estrogen and progesterone levels begin to lower. The spiral arteries close up, and blood stops flowing to the lining's surface — the lining is done growing and thickening.

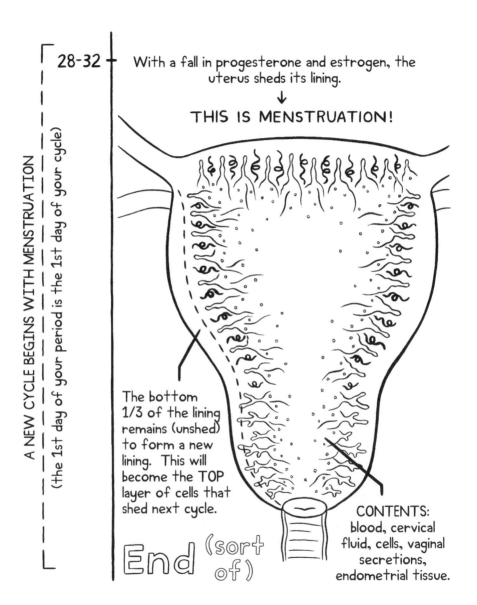

A NEW CYCLE BEGINS WITH MENSTRUATION
(the 1st day of your period is the 1st day of your cycle)

With a fall in progesterone and estrogen, the uterus sheds its lining.

↓

THIS IS MENSTRUATION!

The bottom 1/3 of the lining remains (unshed) to form a new lining. This will become the TOP layer of cells that shed next cycle.

End (sort of)

CONTENTS: blood, cervical fluid, cells, vaginal secretions, endometrial tissue.

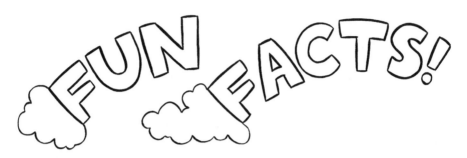

FUN FACTS!

If one ovary is removed, the other one takes over & ovulates every cycle.

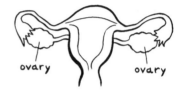

 Ovaries are the size of unshelled almonds! (1 – 1.5 inches)

ACCORDING TO HIPPOCRATES...

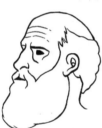

Throat pain = start of menstrual flow.

Nosebleeds = onset of puberty, menstruation, or childbirth (or diverted menstrual blood).

↓

ALSO: "vicarious menstruation" in those whose bleeding was light or infrequent.

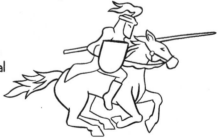

During medieval times, amenorrhea (see p. 26) was treated with vaginal or uterine fumigation (steam often infused with herbs or oils).

14

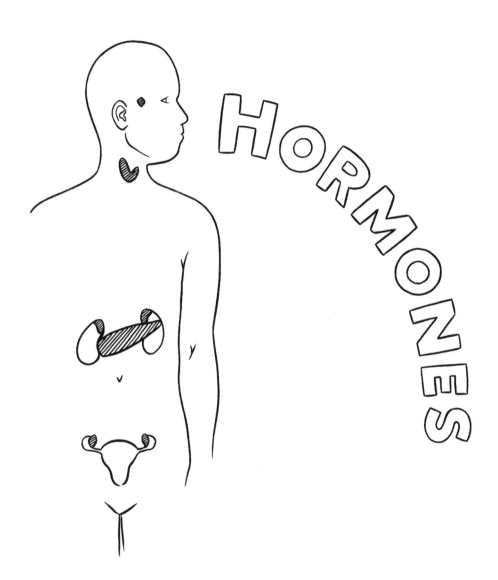

HORMONES

15

hello, hormones

oh, hey.

Hormones are produced by the ovaries & adrenal glands.

Did You Know: estrogen & progesterone keep each other in balance!

PROGESTERONE (P)

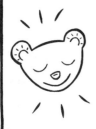

- HELPS you feel content and emotionally balanced.

- REDUCES stress, cramps, muscle weakness, and water retention.

- HELPS your body process sugar and alcohol.

WHEN P LEVELS ARE TOO HIGH

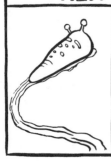

RESULT:

- sluggishness
- low blood sugar
- increased appetite
- muscle aches
- weight gain
- fatigue

- CAUSED BY lack of exercise or poor diet.

ESTROGEN (E)

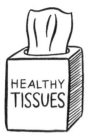

HEALTHY TISSUES

- MAINTAINS healthy skin, tissues, & mucous membranes.

- PRODUCES CHANGES in the ovaries, uterus, fallopian tubes, vagina, & breasts.

- IMPROVES complexion, softens skin, prevents wrinkles, nourishes hair, gives energy.

WHEN E LEVELS ARE TOO HIGH

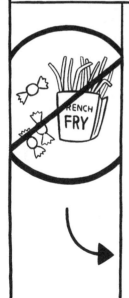

FRENCH FRY

RESULT:

- memory impairment   - insomnia
- sensitive/tingly skin   - anxiety
- water retention

- SLOWS your body's ability to break down fat.

- THROWS OFF blood-sugar levels.

- CONNECTED WITH endometriosis, uterine fibroids, cervical dysplasia, uterine cancer, breast cysts, & breast cancer.

- CAUSED BY stress, fatty or fried foods, sugar, alcohol, meat, & some antidepressants.

YOUR ⇒
ON HORMONAL

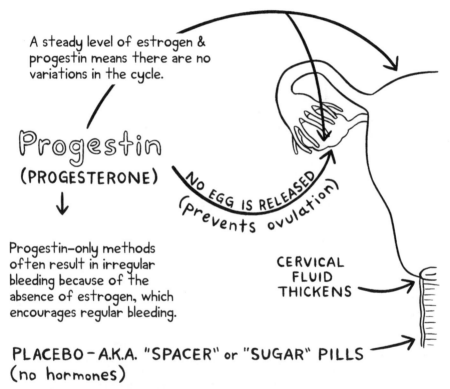

A steady level of estrogen & progestin means there are no variations in the cycle.

Progestin
(PROGESTERONE)
↓

Progestin-only methods often result in irregular bleeding because of the absence of estrogen, which encourages regular bleeding.

NO EGG IS RELEASED
(prevents ovulation)

CERVICAL
FLUID
THICKENS →

PLACEBO – A.K.A. "SPACER" or "SUGAR" PILLS
(no hormones)

When hormones are taken away, the drop in estrogen causes the uterine lining to bleed. (The uterine lining bleeds any time estrogen is suddenly withdrawn from it.)

18

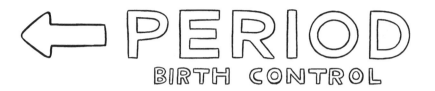

← PERIOD
BIRTH CONTROL

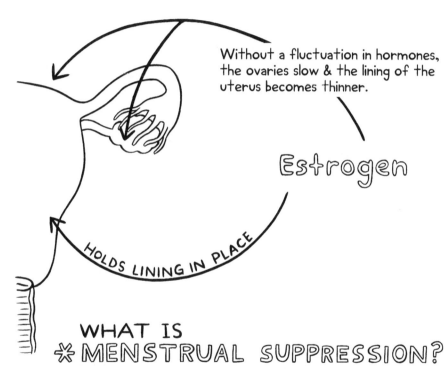

Without a fluctuation in hormones, the ovaries slow & the lining of the uterus becomes thinner.

Estrogen

HOLDS LINING IN PLACE

WHAT IS
✳ MENSTRUAL SUPPRESSION?

Using hormonal birth control to have fewer periods, or to stop bleeding altogether. This is one way of treating problematic or very painful periods. Recently, there is a debate over the idea that regular menstruation is unnatural & should be suppressed. For more information, see the sources on page 66.

PG2 | PROSTAGLANDIN 2

A HORMONE-LIKE SUBSTANCE

Prostaglandins (or PGs) are like hormones. There are different types of prostaglandins that occur naturally throughout your body. Prostaglandin 2 is "pro-inflammatory," which means it causes inflammation (like cramps). PGs also come from fatty acids found in certain foods, so your diet can affect the level of PGs in your body.

CRAMPS → Happen partly because of an increase in PROSTAGLANDIN 2.

Too many prostaglandins = longer, tighter uterine contractions and less oxygen to the muscles.

garlic

Some Things:

These can lower PG levels.

Ginger, flaxseed, garlic, thyme, cinnamon, evening primrose, cloves, hops, and fish oil. (You might already find some of these in your regular diet!)

cloves

Begin taking these around 1 week before menstruation, when PG levels begin to rise. (It can take a few months before you experience changes, so be patient here.)

AVOID: hydrogenated oils, meats, & dairy foods (like cheese). These increase PG levels.

20

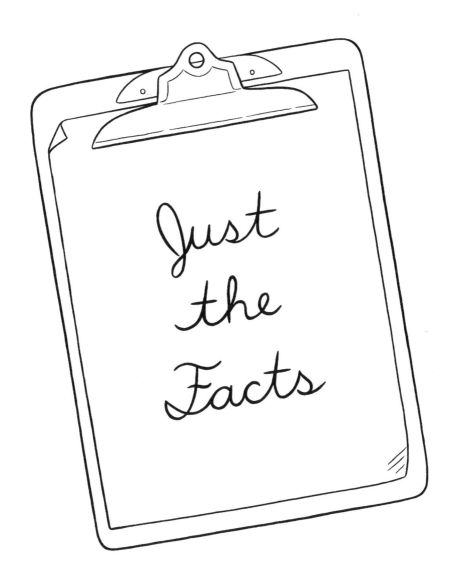

Just the Facts

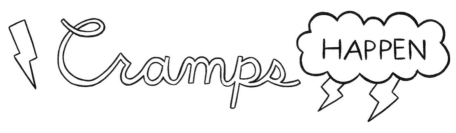

WHAT IS A CRAMP?

Cramps happen when the muscles supporting the uterus contract to help menstrual blood go through the cervical canal and opening.

THE TECHNICAL TERM FOR SEVERE CRAMPS IS "DYSMENORREA."

CAUSES:

Stress, alcohol, a drop in calcium right before menstruation, & excess production of prostaglandins in the uterus. ANTICIPATION can also make cramps worse.

FEEL BETTER:

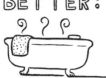

Read through this book and you'll find all kinds of ways to relieve cramps, including yoga, herbal remedies, and dietary changes.

*Don't forget about stress – take a bath, meditate, or just relax.

BONUS TIP:

+100%

Studies show that your pain threshold increases by over 100% from the uterine contractions and release of endorphins that happen at orgasm. It's not a permanent solution, but it can ease cramping and help you relax.

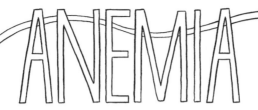

ANEMIA

Anemia is caused by an iron deficiency (meaning there's not enough iron in your blood).

– Anemia is often linked with menstruation.
– People who experience HEAVY menstruation frequently have anemia.

Signs: dizzy, weak, pale, tired most of the time, fall asleep easily, heart palpitations, headaches, digestive problems, listlessness.

Things: (These are iron-rich or increase iron absorption.)

HERBS: burdock root, dandelion, sarsparilla.

FOODS: carrots, green veggies, cumin, parsley, mint, beets, anise.

AVOID: black tea (it slows iron absorption)

➔ Some iron supplements are less effective, or have bad side effects like constipation & stomach problems. They can also block the absorption of vitamin E.

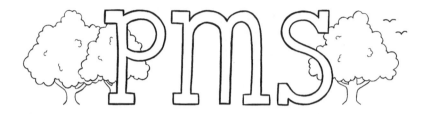

PMS stands for Premenstrual Syndrome. A syndrome is a collection of sensations, signs, or symptoms that occur together.

Some people prefer to use a different term for the menstrual changes they experience – you might like to do this too. For many, the term PMS does not reflect their experience of cycling.

why not PMS?

PMS is not an illness, but the term *syndrome* implies just that (such as Toxic Shock Syndrome). After all, the idea of a syndrome began and continues to be used for diagnosing diseases. Elsewhere, PMS is referred to as a "condition," also suggesting illness or abnormality.

why not illness?

When your body is operating as it is specially designed to (and as the bodies of over half the human population also operate), this cannot be called an illness or condition. This is called healthy.

Your body is a natural habitat, and it functions and fluctuates according to the changes it undergoes. If your habitat is thrown out of balance, there are many simple approaches to restoring that balance.

Here are some common changes & sensations you may experience around menstruation:

sensations:

PLEASANT
creative energy, relief, release, wider range of emotions, increased sex drive, relaxation, connection with body and nature, more intense orgasms, rest, new beginning.

UNCOMFORTABLE
fatigue, mood changes, backache, breast tenderness, cramps, depression, bloating, headache.

some causes:

· Your progesterone levels, along with calcium & magnesium, begin to fall around 3-8 days before menstruation, contributing to cramps and other sensations.

· At the same time, PG2 (Prostaglandin 2) levels increase.

· Stress, lack of sleep &/or exercise, poor diet, alcohol, and hormonal contraceptives can intensify the uncomfortable sensations.

rebalancing:

Adjusting your diet, exercising, and reducing stress levels are all important way of rebalancing. Herbal remedies and yoga can be helpful as well.

Irregularities
& ENDOMETRIOSIS

VERY HEAVY BLEEDING
(menorrhagia)

TAKE MORE
IRON TO PREVENT
ANEMIA

POSSIBLE CAUSES:

- didn't ovulate
- under a lot of stress
- using an intrauterine device
  (IUD)
- having a miscarriage
- fibroids or tumor in uterus

VERY LIGHT or SKIPPED PERIOD
(amenorrhea)

CHANGE
STUFF!

MORE: FIBER;
SOY; VITAMINS
A, E, & C.

LESS: ANIMAL
FAT & STRESS.

POSSIBLE CAUSES:

- stress
- emotional factors
- hormone imbalance
- weight loss
- use of hormonal birth control
- heavy athletic activity
- pregnancy
- breast feeding
- menopause
- cysts or tumors

ENDOMETRIOSIS
A hormonal & immune system disease.

WHAT HAPPENS?

Tissues like the ones that line your uterus grow OUTSIDE the uterus (in the abdomen, on the ovaries, fallopian tubes, and elsewhere).

WHY IS IT A PROBLEM?

Just like the tissues lining the uterus, these tissues respond to hormonal changes, but at menstruation they cannot be shed like those inside the uterus. These tissues have no way of leaving the body.

RESULT:

Inflammation, internal bleeding, scar tissue, infertility, and sometimes other problems. Endometriosis also brings a higher risk for cancer & autoimmune diseases (like lupus, for example).

SYMPTOMS:

Heavy bleeding, severe cramps, pain before & during menstruation, pain during sexual activity, fatigue, and sometimes an increase in allergies, asthma, and eczema.

→ Sometimes endometriosis is mistaken or confused with other disorders.

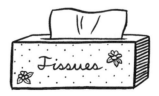

TREATMENT:

It depends on your symptoms, the severity, your age, and other factors.

OPTIONS include:

- hormonal treatment (this stops menstruation & the ovaries from producing estrogen)
- alternative medicine (acupuncture, herbal remedies, etc.)
- surgery

➤ Check p. 68 for info on the Endometriosis Assocation.

THE DIOXIN LINK

Dioxin is a chemical by-product of paper & wood processing, and is also found in food and the environment (due to pesticides, herbicides, and other pollution).

Dioxin builds up in your body, because it gets stored in body fat and your body can't get rid of it.

Dioxin disrupts hormones and is toxic to the immune system. It is believed to be linked with endometriosis, among other health problems, in people of any sex.

In 1992, dioxin received a lot of attention when the FDA discovered trace amounts of the toxin in tampons (due to the process of chlorine-bleaching the material).

The dioxin debate is complex. To learn more, please visit www.zoo-mouse-key.com/dioxin.html.

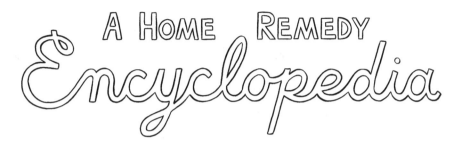

A HOME REMEDY Encyclopedia

Herbal remedies (also called "home remedies" because they can be made at home) can provide a natural and holistic approach to health and healing.

DIFFERENT WAYS TO USE HERBS:

INFUSION: steep herbs and flowers in hot water for 5–20 minutes. The most common infusion is herbal tea.

DECOCTION: boil roots, stems, and bark (the heartier parts of the plant) in water for 5–20 minutes or more.

TINCTURE: combine a large amount of the fresh or dried herb with vinegar (or vodka) in a jar and let steep for 2 days to 2 weeks. This makes a concentrated dose of the herb that is usually taken diluted with water.

POULTICE: a clump of the herb that is heated or moistened, placed directly on the body. You can also wrap it in some thin cloth or cheesecloth.

COMPRESS: a cloth soaked in an infusion or tincture.

GINGER

Ginger has sedative properties that have a relaxing effect on the uterus. It helps with pain, cramps, fatigue, and low libido.

Ginger also regulates the menstrual cycle and encourages delayed menstruation (period inducer).

Make a tea or poultice and apply directly to the abdomen.

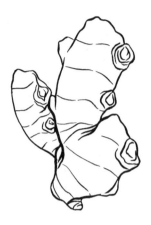

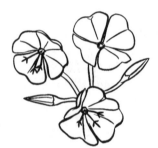

EVENING PRIMROSE

Evening Primrose is usually taken as an oil to treat breast soreness, endometriosis, premenstrual changes, menstrual pain, and cramps.

RED RASPBERRY

Red Raspberry relieves uterine pain and cramps, and treats heavy periods by slowing & reducing bleeding. It also strengthens the uterus and reduces inflammation.

➜ Check with your health care provider if you are pregnant.

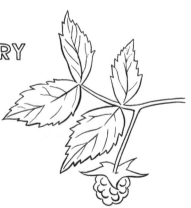

CHASTEBERRY

(Also called Vitex Berry.)

Chasteberry helps to balance hormones*.
It treats irregular cycles, heavy periods,
premenstrual changes, endometriosis,
and cramps.

*Could interfere with hormonal birth control
& hormone replacement therapy.

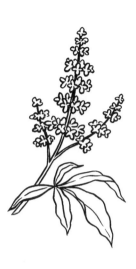

CHAMOMILE

Chamomile's mild sedative properties ease
breast soreness, cramps, and premenstrual
changes (and can help you sleep). It
encourages delayed menstruation and
relaxes the uterus.

MOTHERWORT

Motherwort relaxes the uterus and
relieves cramps, premenstrual changes,
and irregular cycles. It reduces
inflammation & encourages delayed
menstruation.

→ AVOID if pregnant or nursing.

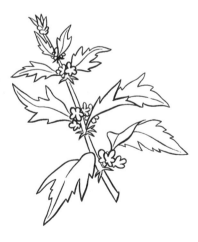

GINKGO

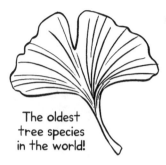

The oldest tree species in the world!

Ginkgo is used to treat premenstrual changes, irregular cycles, headaches & migraines, and fatigue. It improves blood flow throughout the body, as well as libido.

→ AVOID if taking MAOIs for depression.

CINNAMON

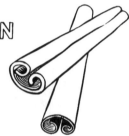

Cinnamon helps ease menstrual pain, cramps, and irregular cycles. It also contains sedative properties that relax the uterus.

DON QUAI

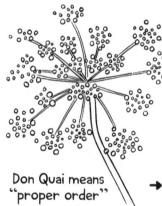

Don Quai means "proper order"

(Also called Chinese Angelica.)

Don Quai relaxes muscles & improves blood flow to the uterus and surrounding area. It helps with irregular cycles, cramps, menstrual pain, premenstrual changes, menopause, and low libido. It also boosts the immune system and encourages delayed menstruation.

→ DO NOT take if you are pregnant, have heavy periods, endometriosis or uterine fibroids.

BLACK COHOSH

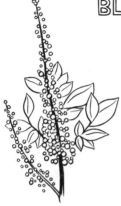

An isoflavone in Black Cohosh acts like a mild estrogen in your body. It treats irregular cycles, premenstrual changes, cramps, excessive bleeding, and menopause.

➜ Be careful using for extended periods of time (6+ months). DO NOT take if you are pregnant or nursing.

OATS

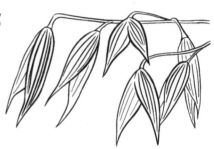

Oats reduce cramps with the muscle-relaxing minerals calcium & magnesium. They also contain mild sedative properties that have a relaxing effect on the uterus.

CRAMP BARK

(Also called Black Haw.)

Cramp Bark reduces inflammation and eases cramps, irregular cycles, and heavy bleeding.

Infusion: 2 cups boiling water plus 1 tsp. shredded or ground cramp bark. Steep for 30 minutes. Makes a 2-day supply. Take 1/3 cup twice daily. Keep refrigerated.

33

Home Remedy
FUN FACTS

The most popular herbal supplement (or drug) in the U.S. is COFFEE.

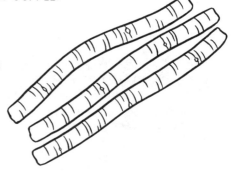

The LIVER helps to clear excess estrogen from your body. A healthy liver will keep estrogen levels balanced. (A good herb for the liver is Burdock Root.)

If you experience cramps, anxiety, or irritability, avoid drinking COFFEE. It prevents your body from absorbing calcium, magnesium, iron, and other nutrients.

Rub your belly with a massage oil made with SAGE essential oil to slow heavy menstrual bleeding.

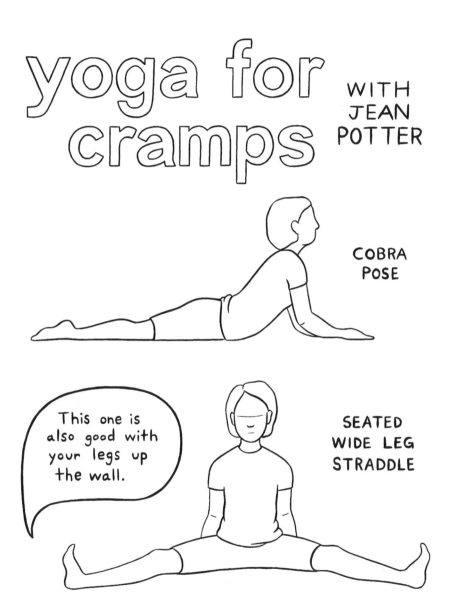

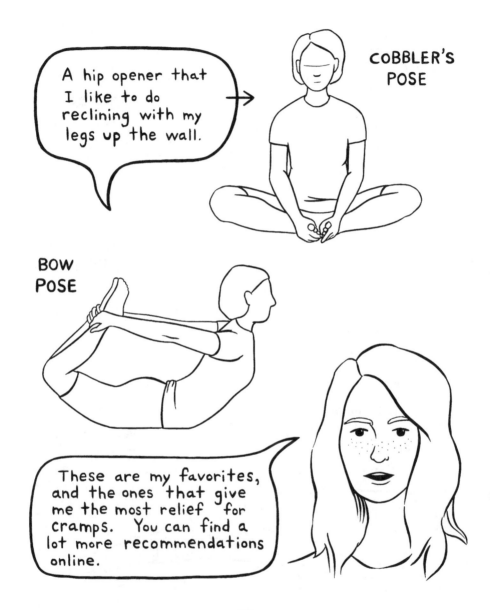

A hip opener that I like to do reclining with my legs up the wall.

COBBLER'S POSE

BOW POSE

These are my favorites, and the ones that give me the most relief for cramps. You can find a lot more recommendations online.

HOW IT WORKS

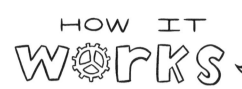

How to use products and other exciting info

The term *product* refers to anything that is used for catching menstrual flow, whether it's handmade, commercial, alternative or mainstream.

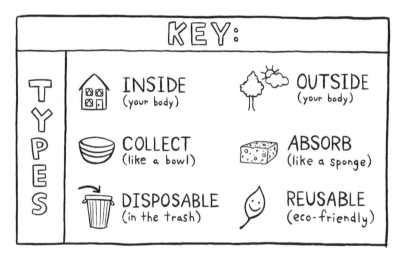

KEY:

TYPES

INSIDE (your body)

OUTSIDE (your body)

COLLECT (like a bowl)

ABSORB (like a sponge)

DISPOSABLE (in the trash)

REUSABLE (eco-friendly)

OTHER FACTORS

 ORGANIC

 ALL-COTTON

 CHLORINE-FREE

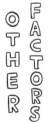

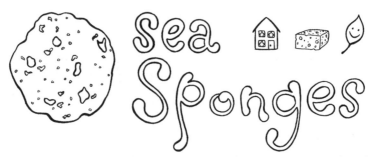

Sea Sponges

→ Change (remove & rinse) every 4–8 hours.

→ Rest in the upper vagina.

HOW TO INSERT: wet sponge & squeeze out the extra water. Insert with your fingers. Your sponge should feel comfortable.

HOW TO REMOVE: use your fingers OR sew a piece of string or (unflavored) dental floss to the sponge to use like a tampon string.

HOW TO CLEAN: remove your sponge & rinse it at least 4 times per day. DO NOT USE SOAP — this will upset the natural pH balance of your vagina.

BETWEEN CYCLES: if desired, you can rinse your sponge in a vinegar/water or baking soda/water solution. Either way, let it air dry then store in a cool, dry place.

*You can also BOIL your sponge between cycles for 5–10 minutes. This will kill any bacteria. Boiling will make the sponge denser & more absorbent, and will also shrink, toughen, and shorten its lifespan for use.

*Sea sponges may contain pollutants from the ocean (which is polluted).

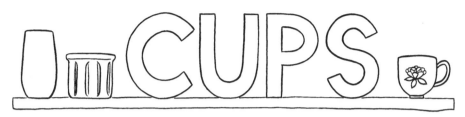 # CUPS

→ Empty a few times per day.

THE KEEPER

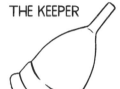

→ Lasts up to 10 years.

→ 2 sizes: regular size (B), & a slightly larger size (A) for those who have given birth (the cup is 1/8" wider).

→ Made of natural rubber (latex).

✳ SILICONE VERSIONS (ideal for those with a latex allergy) include Moon Cup, Diva Cup, and Lunette Cup.

✳ Cups rest in the LOWER VAGINA, so you'll probably feel them more.

Tips: – Trim the pull-tab to a length that's comfortable to you.

– A full bladder can sometimes push the cup out of position, causing a leak.

✳ A DIAPHRAGM or CERVICAL CAP can also be worn like a menstrual cup.

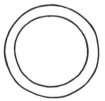 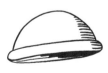

HOW TO INSERT: with clean hands, fold the sides of your cup together. Then fold again.

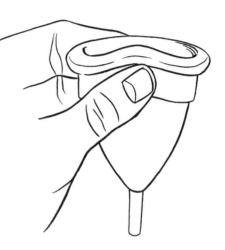

With your body in a comfortable position, insert your cup into your vagina. The cup will unfold when you release your fingers.

Gently rotate your cup slightly, and pull down and forward (also gently) so that it's positioned at your vaginal opening. The stem or pull-tab should be outside your vagina.

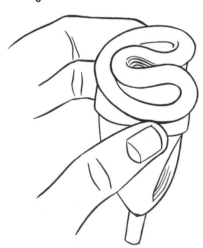

HOW TO REMOVE: sit on the toilet (or in the shower) and pinch the base of the cup with your fingers - this releases the suction that has been holding it in place.

Slowly & gently remove your cup. Rinse and reinsert.

BETWEEN CYCLES: wash your cup in soapy water; rinse thoroughly and let air dry. Store in a cool, dry place- or in the fabric pouch that comes with some cups.

*You can also rinse (not soak) your cup in a vinegar/water solution (1 part vinegar + 9 parts water) for a minute or two. [A higher vinegar solution can damage your cup.]

40

INSTEAD SOFTCUP

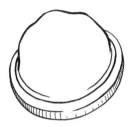

→ One-time use.

→ Can be worn during intercourse.

→ Made of Kraton (a plastic).

→ Can be worn up to 12 hours.

✳ Does NOT protect you from Sexually Transmitted Infections (STIs) or pregnancy.

✳ Not to be confused with a diaphragm, which has a similar shape.

✳ Not recommended for use with an IUD (cup could dislodge the IUD).

– Rests in the UPPER VAGINA, under the cervix.

HOW TO INSERT: fold the cup and insert it into your vagina using your fingers. You should push it back, not up like you would with a tampon.

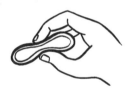

HOW TO REMOVE: use your middle finger (or whatever finger works best for you) to gently hook under the rim of your cup. To avoid spilling, keep your cup level with the floor.

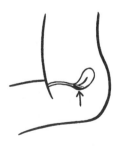

✳ DO NOT flush your softcup. Wrap it in tissue & throw in the trash.

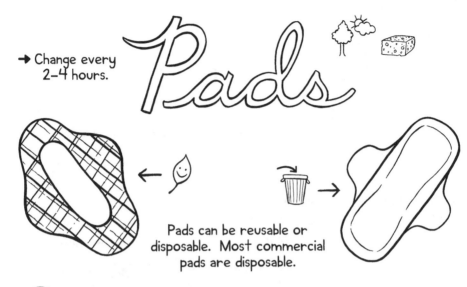

→ Change every 2-4 hours.

Pads

Pads can be reusable or disposable. Most commercial pads are disposable.

DEODORIZED pads are associated with yeast infections (and they promote the idea that you are dirty & smelly– which you're not). Don't use them.

More & more people are choosing CLOTH pads, because they're better for the environment, are often more comfortable, and they tend to look pretty awesome.

PIMPs (Party In My Pants), Luna Pads, and Glad Rags are some companies that make reusable cloth pads.

MAKE YOUR OWN with towels, old t-shirts, or any cotton cloth.

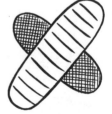

Look on the internet or in the Sources & Resources section for a link to d.i.y. instructions!

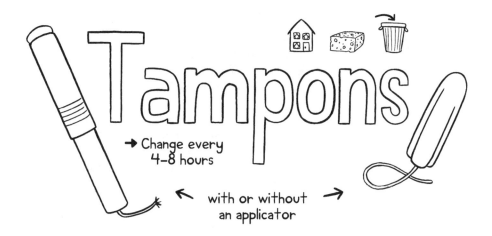

Tampons

→ Change every 4-8 hours

← with or without → an applicator

 ALL-COTTON tampons are recommended. They're safer than rayon tampons because there is a lower risk of TSS.

 ORGANIC & CHLORINE-FREE are recommended because they are free of chemical residues that could irritate your vagina.

 DEODORIZED tampons can cause yeast infections (and they promote the idea that you are dirty & smelly — which you're not). Don't use them.

✱ Tampons rest in the UPPER VAGINA, so you'll probably feel them less.

✱ Tampons are not really flushable. Wrap them in tissue & throw in the trash.

HOW TO INSERT: if you've never used a tampon before, start with one that has an applicator and the lowest absorbency. It's also easier to insert a tampon when your flow is on the heavier side. When your bleeding is light, it can be more difficult.

Sit, stand, or squat in a comfortable position. Hold the tampon near the middle (most tampons have helpful little lines here), where the two tubes meet. Use your free hand to part your labia, and place the tip of your tampon at your vaginal opening.

→ A mirror can help you find your vaginal opening! See also the drawing on page 6.

Now gently push the tampon in. (Note: don't start pushing the inner tube into the outer tube yet! You're just inserting the outer tube into your vagina right now.) Imagine aiming for your lower back.

Once the outer tube is all the way inside you, use your index finger to push the inner tube into the outer tube. This pushes the tampon the rest of the way into your vagina. Neat, huh? (Note: the inner tube needs to go all the way into the outer tube.)

Now you can remove the applicator.

Is the string outside your vagina where you can reach it? Good, you'll use that later (see next page).

OUTER TUBE

INNER TUBE

HOW TO REMOVE: relax your pelvic and vaginal muscles, and tug on the string of your tampon. It should remove easily. If it's difficult or uncomfortable to remove, use a lower absorbency next time. (If your flow is very light, consider using a cloth or pad instead, or nothing at all.)

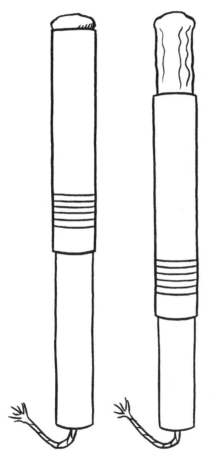

Note: If your tampon is inserted correctly, you shouldn't be able to feel it; you should feel comfortable. If you're uncomfortable, remove your tampon, throw it out, and try again with a new one.

➜ For non-applicator tampons, use your fingers to insert, and one or two fingertips to guide the tampon into place.

Tips!

For easier insertion, try putting a little personal lubricant (like KY or Astroglide) on the tip of your tampon.

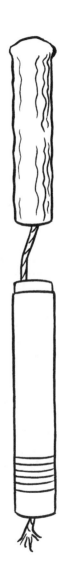

45

WHAT EXACTLY IS

TSS?

TOXIC SHOCK SYNDROME

When you buy tampons, you'll find a warning inside the box that talks about TSS. Toxic Shock Syndrome (or TSS) is a serious but uncommon blood infection. Because it is life-threatening, it's important for you to know about it. You may have also heard about a lot of people having TSS in the 1980s. Today, it's not something you need to worry too much about – just make sure to change your tampons regularly, and use an absorbency that's right for you.

Toxic Shock is caused by a toxin released by staph bacteria, a bacteria present in about 10% of healthy vaginas. Staph bacteria can also be introduced by fingers inserting a tampon, cup, or other menstrual device.

All types of people can contract TSS in various ways – it is not just menstruation related.

SIGNS & SYMPTOMS: high fever, drop in blood pressure, vomiting, diarrhea, sunburn-like rash, severe muscle ache and weakness.

BACTERIA

If you have questions about TSS, look up more information about it or talk with your health care provider.

1980:

Before the 80s, the link between TSS and tampons was relatively unknown. In 1980, a rise in TSS cases led to an investigation by the Centers for Disease Control & Prevention. As a result, tampon safety regulations were put into place, including Absorbency Ratings, warnings, and instructions for safest use on packaging.

Q: Could a TSS outbreak happen again?

No – it's incredibly unlikely. The incident in 1980 happened because TSS was not yet a concern. In fact, the term 'TSS' did not exist until 1978! There were no absorbency ratings or warnings on tampon packaging like we see today.

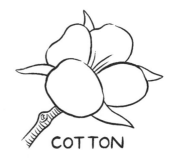
COTTON

Part of what led to the outbreak in 1980 was a growing demand for more absorbent tampons, including a tampon that could "contain an entire menstrual flow without leaking or replacement." Manufacturers turned to synthetic fibers, which were more absorbent (before that most tampons were cotton).

RAYON

It turns out all synthetic fibers amplify the TSS toxin (cotton does not).

TODAY:
- Tampon absorbency is HALF of what it used to be.

- 3 of the 4 synthetic fibers used in tampons in 1980 have been removed (viscose rayon remains).

HISTORY, Traditions, and Folklore

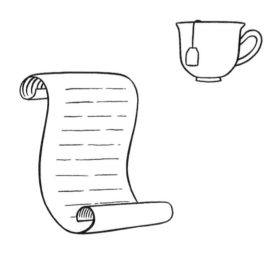

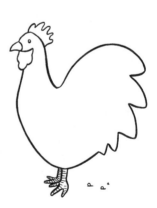

Presenting the

HISTORY

of PRODUCTS ®™

(IN A TIMELINE!)

Before the industrial era and the advent of commercial wares, menstrual products were not widely available like they are today.

Items to absorb, hold, or catch menstrual blood were made by hand for 1,000s of years (ever since people began menstruating, that is). These items were often very similar to today's tampons, cups, and pads.

In the late 1800s, industrialization really took off. The result: mass-produced and ready-made menstrual products that were widely available. No more need to make your own!

Recently, there has been a renewed interest in hand-made menstrual gear, or natural, organic, and reuseable products.

Plants and natural fibers have always been a preferred method for catching or absorbing menstrual blood.

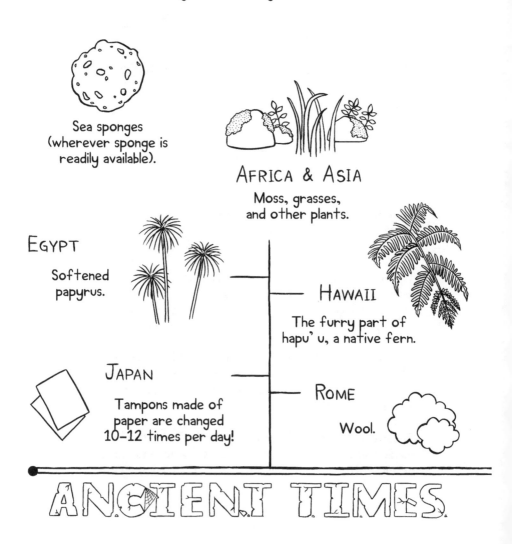

Sea sponges (wherever sponge is readily available).

AFRICA & ASIA

Moss, grasses, and other plants.

EGYPT

Softened papyrus.

HAWAII

The furry part of hapu' u, a native fern.

JAPAN

Tampons made of paper are changed 10–12 times per day!

ROME

Wool.

ANCIENT TIMES

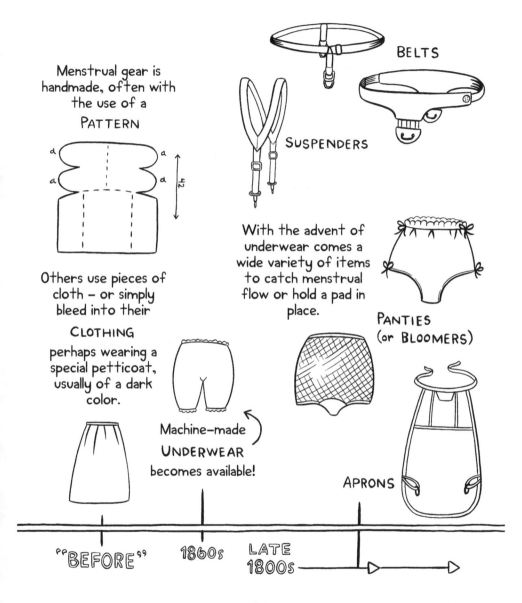

Menstrual gear is handmade, often with the use of a PATTERN

Others use pieces of cloth - or simply bleed into their CLOTHING perhaps wearing a special petticoat, usually of a dark color.

BELTS

SUSPENDERS

With the advent of underwear comes a wide variety of items to catch menstrual flow or hold a pad in place.

PANTIES (or BLOOMERS)

Machine-made UNDERWEAR becomes available!

APRONS

"BEFORE"   1860s   LATE 1800s

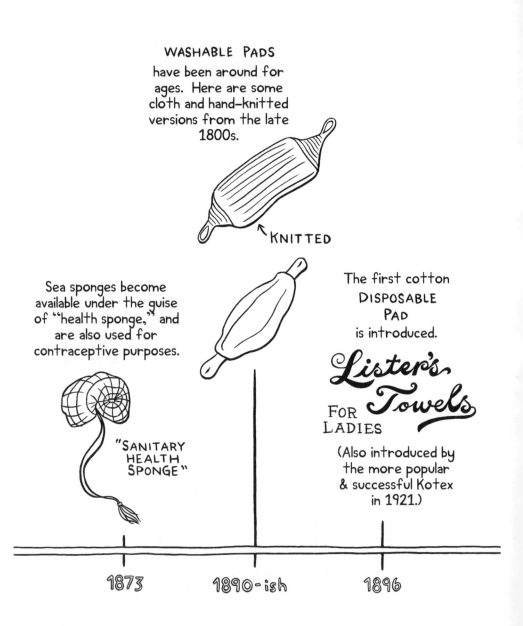

WASHABLE PADS have been around for ages. Here are some cloth and hand-knitted versions from the late 1800s.

← KNITTED

Sea sponges become available under the guise of "health sponge," and are also used for contraceptive purposes.

"SANITARY HEALTH SPONGE"

The first cotton DISPOSABLE PAD is introduced.

Lister's Towels

FOR LADIES

(Also introduced by the more popular & successful Kotex in 1921.)

1873   1890-ish   1896

52

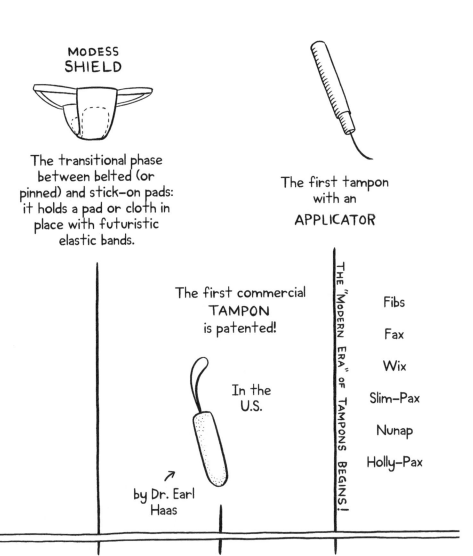

MODESS
SHIELD

The transitional phase between belted (or pinned) and stick-on pads: it holds a pad or cloth in place with futuristic elastic bands.

The first tampon
with an
APPLICATOR

The first commercial
TAMPON
is patented!

In the
U.S.

by Dr. Earl
Haas

THE "MODERN ERA" OF TAMPONS BEGINS!

Fibs

Fax

Wix

Slim-Pax

Nunap

Holly-Pax

mid-1920s   1933   1936

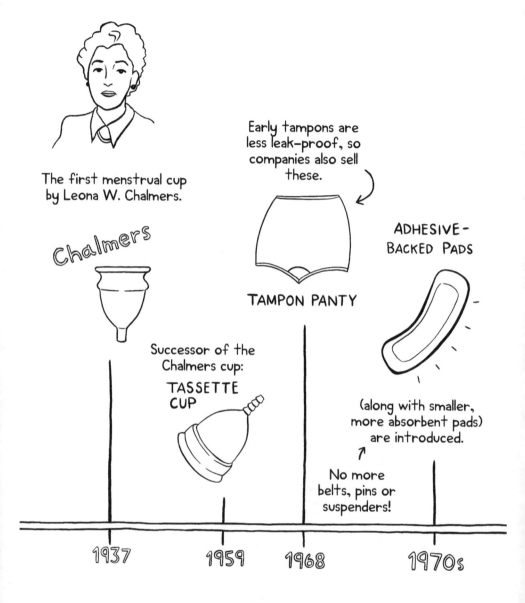

The first menstrual cup by Leona W. Chalmers.

Chalmers

Early tampons are less leak-proof, so companies also sell these.

TAMPON PANTY

ADHESIVE-BACKED PADS

Successor of the Chalmers cup:
TASSETTE CUP

(along with smaller, more absorbent pads) are introduced.

No more belts, pins or suspenders!

1937   1959   1968   1970s

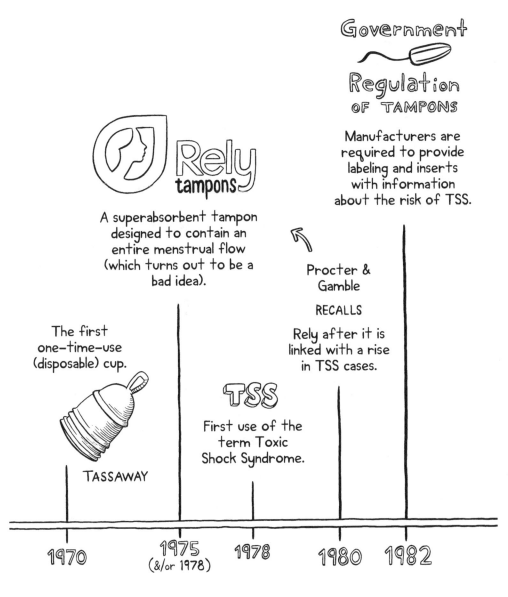

Government

Regulation
OF TAMPONS

Manufacturers are
required to provide
labeling and inserts
with information
about the risk of TSS.

Rely
tampons

A superabsorbent tampon
designed to contain an
entire menstrual flow
(which turns out to be a
bad idea).

Procter &
Gamble

RECALLS

Rely after it is
linked with a rise
in TSS cases.

The first
one-time-use
(disposable) cup.

TSS

First use of the
term Toxic
Shock Syndrome.

TASSAWAY

1970

1975
(&/or 1978)

1978

1980

1982

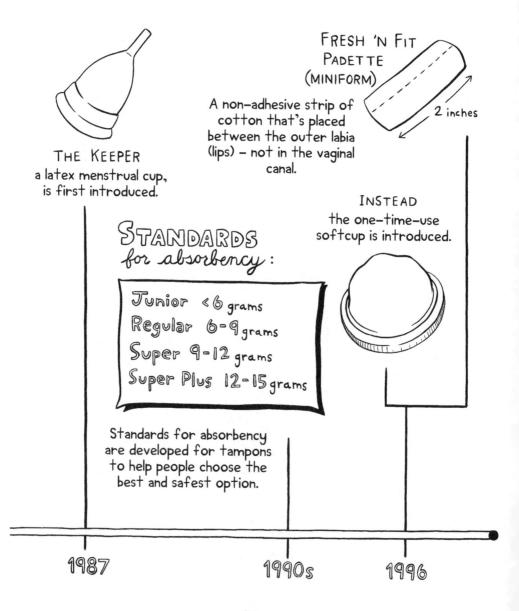

THE KEEPER
a latex menstrual cup, is first introduced.

FRESH 'N FIT PADETTE (MINIFORM)

A non-adhesive strip of cotton that's placed between the outer labia (lips) – not in the vaginal canal.

2 inches

STANDARDS for absorbency :

Junior	< 6 grams
Regular	6 - 9 grams
Super	9 - 12 grams
Super Plus	12 - 15 grams

Standards for absorbency are developed for tampons to help people choose the best and safest option.

INSTEAD
the one-time-use softcup is introduced.

1987   1990s   1996

Menotoxin
know your poison

Menotoxin means "menstrual poison." It refers to a poison or toxin that was once believed to be present in menstrual blood, and the ability of a menstruating person to cause harm. This belief originated thousands of years ago, and is typically regarded today as folklore.

The following are some examples of things that would, according to myth, spoil if exposed to someone who was menstruating.

It's hard to say who created these beliefs: non-menstruators who felt intimidated by monthly bleeding, or menstruators seeking a break from their labors.

Mayonnaise is
unsuccessful.

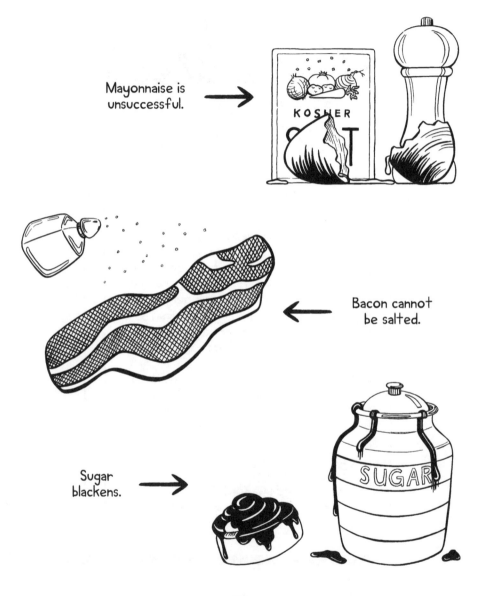

Bacon cannot
be salted.

Sugar
blackens.

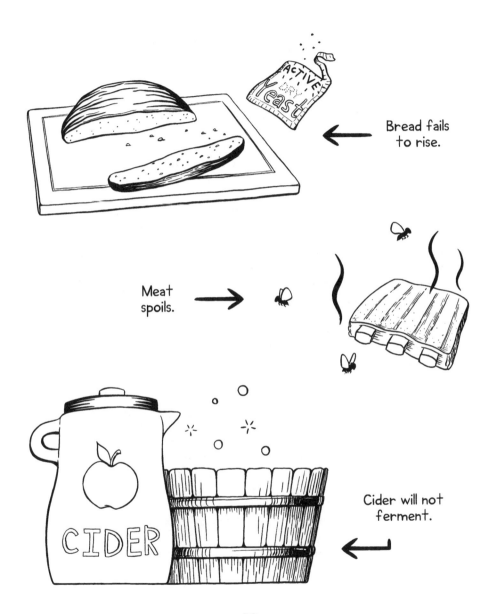

Bread fails
to rise.

Meat
spoils.

Cider will not
ferment.

59

FUN WITH ETYMOLOGY

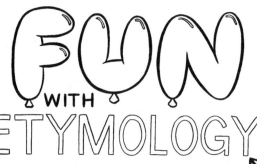

↖ The history of a word.

Estrogen

estrus + –gen

estrus: 1850, from Latin *oestrus* "frenzy, gadfly," from Greek *oistros* "gadfly, breeze, sting, mad impulse" (related to Lithuanian *aistra* "violent passion," Latin *ira* "anger").

–gen: meaning something that produces or causes.

Testosterone

testis + ster(oid) + –one (chemical ending)

testis: (pl. testes), 1704, from Latin *testis* "testicle," usually regarded as a special application of *testis* "witness" (see testament), presumably because it "bears witness" to virility. The Greek legal sense of *parastates* "supporter, defender" or in the sense of twin "supporting pillars, props of a mast."

steroid: 1936, from Greek *-oeides* "-like," from *eidos* "form, shape."

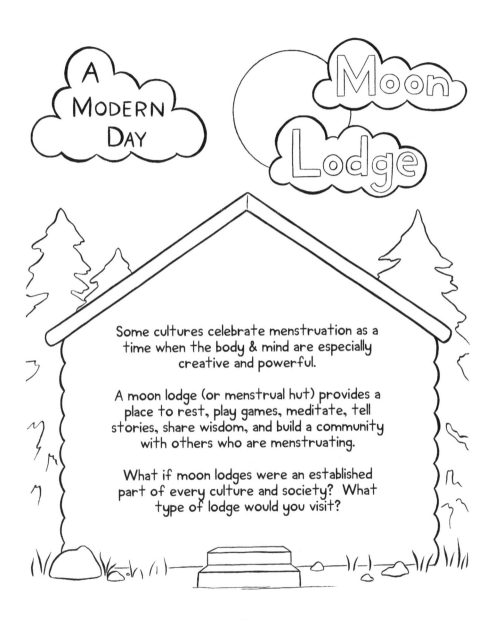

A
MODERN
DAY

Moon

Lodge

Some cultures celebrate menstruation as a time when the body & mind are especially creative and powerful.

A moon lodge (or menstrual hut) provides a place to rest, play games, meditate, tell stories, share wisdom, and build a community with others who are menstruating.

What if moon lodges were an established part of every culture and society? What type of lodge would you visit?

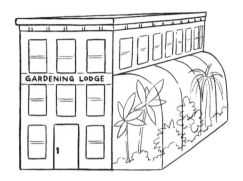

Gardening Lodge:
farming, herbs,
vegetables, flowers.

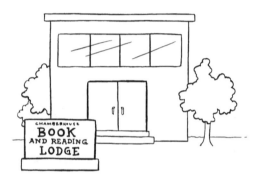

Book & Reading Lodge:
quiet, reading, writing,
book groups.

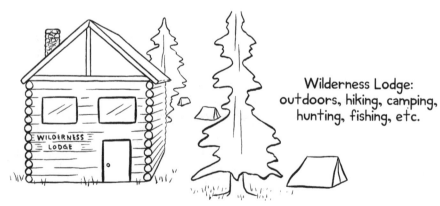

Wilderness Lodge:
outdoors, hiking, camping,
hunting, fishing, etc.

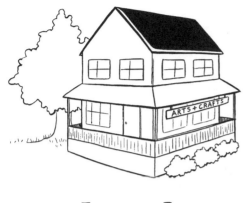

Art & Crafts Lodge:
drawing, printmaking,
sculpture, comic books,
painting, bookbinding,
woodworking, weaving,
jewelry.

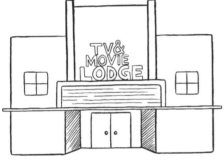

TV & Movie Lodge:
film, video, popcorn,
couches.

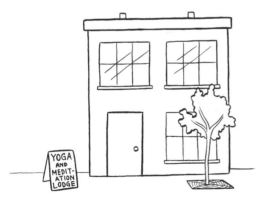

Yoga & Meditation Lodge:
relaxation, meditation,
different kinds of yoga,
deep breathing.

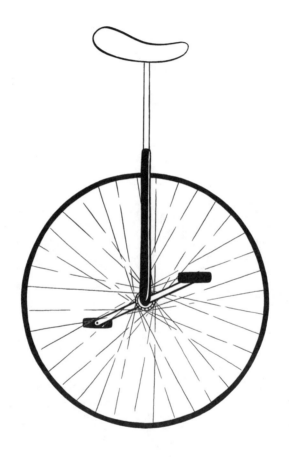

Sources

& RESOURCES

BOOKS

OUR BODIES, OURSELVES, The Boston Women's Health Book Collective, 2005

A NEW VIEW OF A WOMAN'S BODY, The Federation of Feminist Women's Health Centers, 1991

GIRLS IN POWER: GENDER, BODY, AND MENSTRUATION IN ADOLESCENCE, Laura Fingerson, 2006

THE WOMAN IN THE BODY: A CULTURAL ANALYSIS OF REPRODUCTION, Emily Martin, 2001

THE V BOOK: A DOCTOR'S GUIDE TO COMPLETE VULVO-VAGINAL HEALTH, Elizabeth G. Stewart, M.D. and Paula Spencer, 2002

ARE YOU THERE GOD? IT'S ME, MARGARET. Judy Blume, 1970

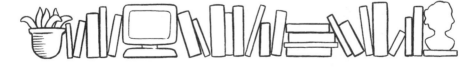

MORE BOOKS

THE CURSE: CONFRONTING THE LAST UNMENTIONABLE TABOO: MENSTRUATION, Karen Houppert, 1999

THE STORY OF V, Catherine Blackledge, 2003

FLOW: THE CULTURAL STORY OF MENSTRUATION, Elissa Stein and Susan Kim, 2009

THE SECOND SEX, Simone de Beauvoir, 1952

CUNT: A DECLARATION OF INDEPENDENCE, Inga Muscio, 2002

HERBS FOR HEALTH AND HEALING: A DRUG-FREE GUIDE TO PREVENTION AND CARE, Kathi Keville, 1996

THE GREEN PHARMACY HERBAL HANDBOOK, James A. Duke, Ph.D., 2000

IS MENSTRUATION OBSOLETE?, Elsimar M. Coutinho with Sheldon J. Segal, 1999

THE BLESSINGS OF THE CURSE: NO MORE PERIODS?, Susan Rako, M.D., 2006

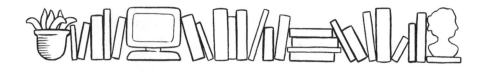

FILM

PERIOD: THE END OF MENSTRUATION, Giovanna Chesler, 2005 (www.periodthemovie.com)

ARTICLES

"THE QUESTION'S ABSORBING: 'ARE TAMPONS LITTLE WHITE LIES?',"" Joanna Citrinbaum, The Daily Collegian, October 14, 2003

"JOHN ROCK'S ERROR," Malcolm Gladwell, The New Yorker, March 13, 2000

"MS. TAMPON GOES TO WASHINGTON: THE DIOXIN CONTROVERSY," Estronaut: A Forum For Women's Health, 1999 <<http://www.estronaut.com/a/dioxin_tampons.htm>>

"HOW THE INFLAMMATORY SYSTEM WORKS." <<http://www.drmurphreestore.com/arthritisandpain.html>> August 18, 2010 (Prostaglandins)

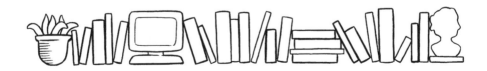

WEB

Museum of Menstruation and Women's Health:
www.mum.org

Scarleteen (Sex Positive Sex Education):
www.scarleteen.com

Feminist Women's Health Centers: www.fwhc.org

LGBT Health Channel:
http://lgbthealth.healthcommunities.com

Our Bodies, Ourselves: www.ourbodiesourselves.org

Go Ask Alice! – Columbia University's Health Q&A Service:
www.goaskalice.columbia.edu

The Endometriosis Association: www.endometriosisassn.org

Online Etymology Dictionary: www.etymonline.com

OTHER

Reusable Menstrual Products (and instructions to make
your own!): www.ecomenses.com

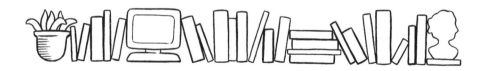